Nature's Recipe Grain Free Cookbook

Many Deliciously Easy Grain Free Recipes that will Keep You Known for Tasty Yet Healthy Treats

Table of Contents

Introduction 4

    Chia-Orange-Chocolate Breakfast Parfait 6

    Veggie Egg Cups 9

    Banana Flour Waffles 11

    Grain-Free Breakfast Burrito 13

    Applesauce Grain-Free Pancakes 15

    Spiced Carrots & Cauliflower 17

    No-Grain Chilaquiles 19

    Red Lentil Soup 22

    Crème Fraiche Carrots & Apricots 25

    Creamy Tomato Soup 28

    Shrimp Ceviche 30

    Slow-Cooker Pork 32

    Herbed Braised Beans 34

    Lemon-Kissed Bean Salad 37

    Mango Chicken Salad 39

    Broccoli & Roast Salmon 41

    Shrimp with Grits 44

    Chili Gremolata Roasted Shrimp 47

    Steak Vinaigrette with Vegetables 50

    Southwestern Style Squash Soup 53

    Lemon Chicken with Veggies 56

Kelp Noodles with Sesame 59

Ham & White Bean Slow Cooker Soup 61

Asian Vegetable Stir Fry 64

Grain-Free Potatoes & Roast Chicken 67

Pumpkin Roll Cake 69

Grain-Free Honey Cake 73

Peach Cobbler 75

Apple-Cinnamon Grain-Free Cake 78

Grain-Free Chocolate Cake 80

Conclusion 83

Introduction

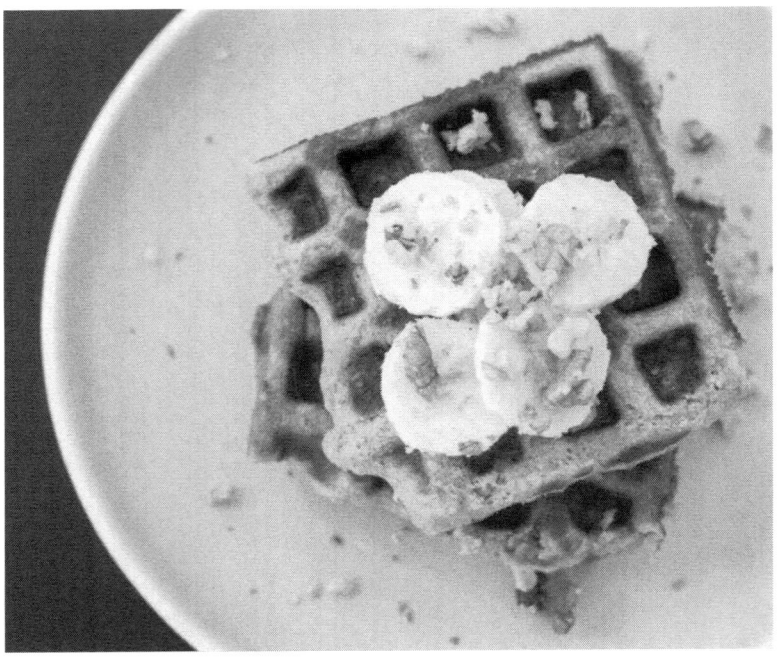

Why would anyone even think of serving grain free dishes in their household?

Physicians have oftentimes diagnosed medical problems as a result of the consumption of grains. In this cookbook, the recipes have by-passed gluten-free recipes since all grains have been eliminated, to include, oats, rice and corn.

Some grains have been linked to the unhealthy occurrence of inflammation in the body, which often leads to various health issues such as diverse colon disorders, leaky gut syndrome, autoimmune disorders and chronic diseases.

Many persons have problems with wheat consumption as they find it hard to digest. If you have a problem with the consumption of gluten, most likely, you should not be consuming grains either. Consumption of grains sometimes leads to weight gain and insulin resistance.

These recipes are geared to ease or eliminate any issues you might have with digestion, will balance both good and bad bacteria found in the gut and will assist in the relief of inflammation in your body. You stand a good chance to lose those negative effects which are caused by eating heavily processed and refined grains. Positive results can be attained if you choose a grain free diet.

Chia-Orange-Chocolate Breakfast Parfait

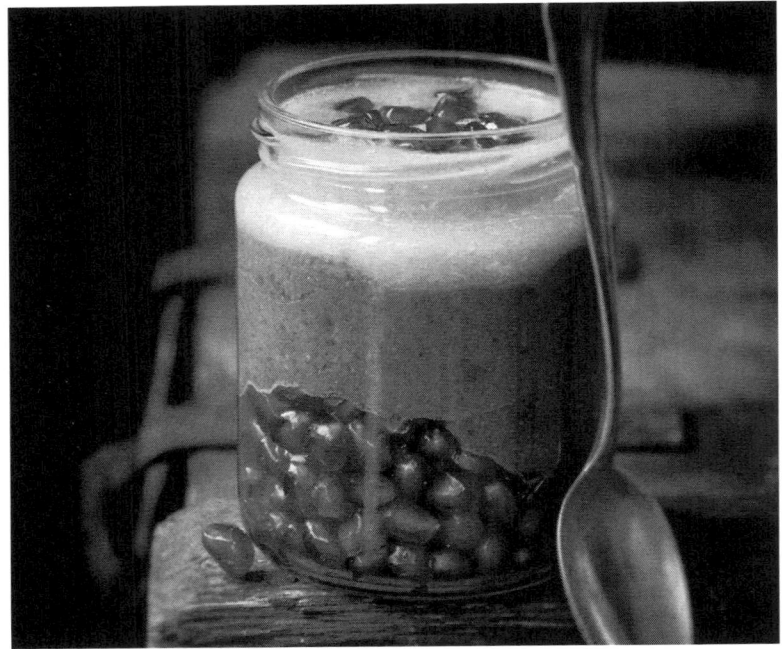

This vegan breakfast is made with non-dairy milk and dates, blended to create a healthy and creamy meal. There are no grains used, and the dish is flavored with oranges and pomegranates.

Serves: 2

Time: 10 minutes + 4-8 hours setting time

Ingredients:

- 2 cups of coconut milk, non-dairy
- 6 tbsp. of chia
- 6 tbsp. of cacao
- 1/2 cup of pitted dates, soft
- 2 oranges, zest only
- 1 tsp. of cinnamon, ground
- 2 peeled, blended oranges, fresh
- 1 cup of pomegranate seeds

Directions:

1. To prepare orange topping, place peeled oranges in blender. Pulse till it shows you a thick textured juice. It thickens more when refrigerated. Add 1 tsp. of honey, as desired.

2. Pour milk in a medium container and add chia. Refrigerate for four hours or more, or overnight, so pudding will set completely.

3. Add chia pudding, cinnamon, dates, cacao and orange zest to food processor. Blend till consistency is smooth. Chill for 1/2 hour.

4. To assemble jars, put 1/4 pomegranate seeds as base. Add 1/2 cup chocolate pudding and top with orange sauce. Serve cold.

Veggie Egg Cups

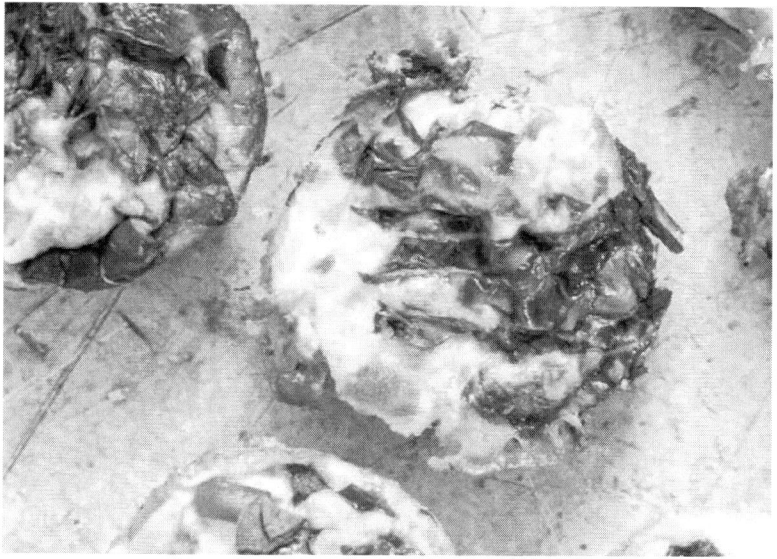

This recipe is for superfood in cups. They're easily made, and you can refrigerate them

for several days and use them for nutritious and convenient to-go breakfasts or snacks.

Serves: 6

Time: 35 minutes

Ingredients:

- 4 eggs, large
- 1/2 bunch of 1/2-inch chunked asparagus
- 1/2 cauliflower with heads removed and florets crumbled
- 1 cup of quartered tomatoes, grape
- 3 chopped green onions
- 1/2 tsp. of garlic powder
- 1 tsp. of oregano, dried

Directions:

1. Preheat the oven to 375F.

2. Pour the eggs into small sized bowl. Add oregano and garlic. Mix by whisking.

3. Portion out the veggies in 6-large muffin cups. Begin with cauliflower.

4. Pour the egg mixture to cover the cups. They should be about 3/4 full.

5. Bake at 375F for 18-20 minutes and serve while warm or chilled.

Banana Flour Waffles

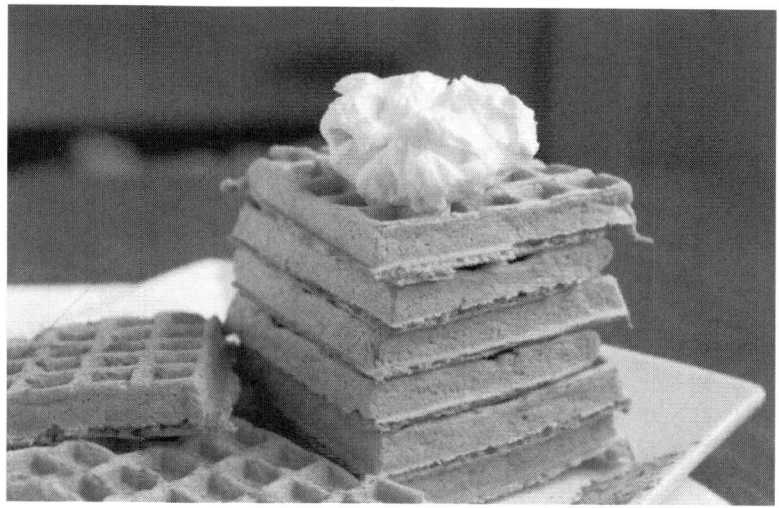

Banana flour is grain free and gluten free, and this recipe also does not include refined sugars. Even kids– who like the sweetest breakfast treats– will love these tasty waffles.

Serves: 6

Time: 25 minutes

Ingredients:

- 1 cup of flour, banana
- 1/3 cup of flour, almond
- 1 tsp. of baking powder

- 1 dash of salt, kosher
- 2 eggs, large
- 2 tbsp. of avocado oil
- 3/4 cup of milk, almond

Directions:

1. Preheat your waffle iron

2. Add dry ingredients to large sized bowl. Blend by whisking.

3. Combine your wet and dry ingredients.

4. Grease waffle iron and cook as usual.

5. Serve with syrup and pecans.

Grain-Free Breakfast Burrito

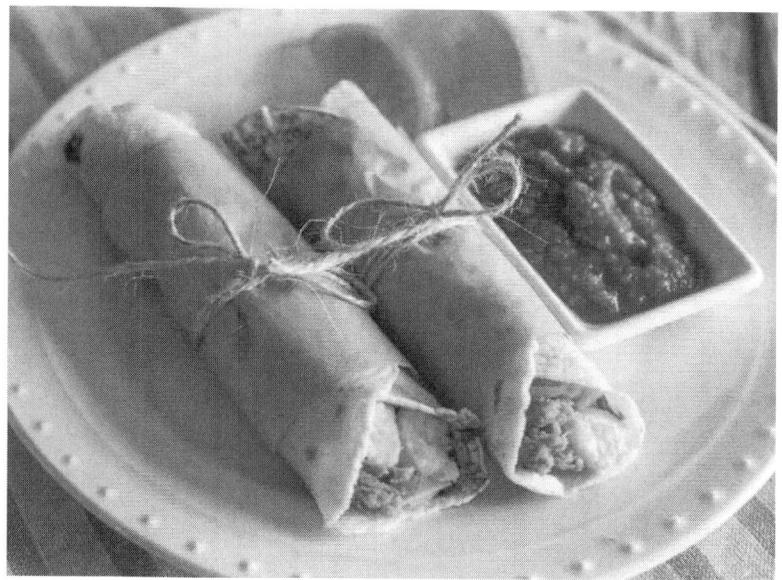

Giving up grain doesn't need to be a drag for you. Grain free foods can be enjoyable. These Paleo breakfast burritos offer great flavor, without flavorless, floppy flour tortillas.

Serves: 2

Time: 10 minutes

Ingredients:

- Sliced ham in large enough pieces to roll
- 4 eggs, whites only

- 1/2 cup of chopped vegetables, your choice
- Optional: cilantro, guacamole, salsa

Directions:

1. Sauté vegetables in small amount of oil on med-high.

2. Whisk eggs in small sized bowl. Pour over vegetables.

3. Scramble mixture in skillet with spatula till cooked completely through. Remove eggs from pan.

4. Roll ham slices around eggs. Return to skillet. Grill for several seconds on each side.

5. Serve with guacamole, salsa, etc., with cilantro to garnish.

Applesauce Grain-Free Pancakes

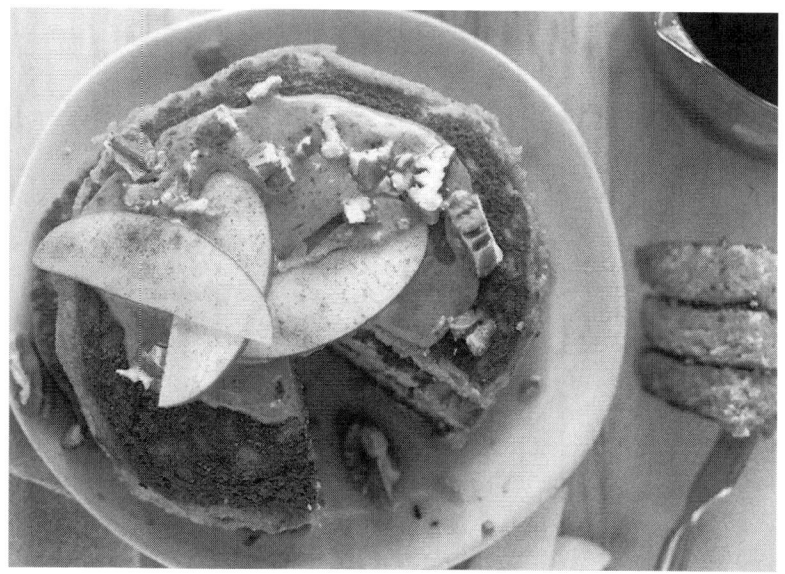

These delicious, grain-free pancakes are made with applesauce instead of grains. This is a high protein breakfast that's also Paleo-friendly and gluten free.

Serves: 5

Time: 1/2 hour

Ingredients:

- 2 large eggs, free-range
- 1/3 cup of unsweetened applesauce

- 1/4 cup of meal, almond
- 1/2 tsp. of baking powder
- 1/4 tsp. of vanilla extract, pure
- 1/2 tbsp. of honey, organic
- Maple syrup

Directions:

1. Whisk the two eggs in small sized bowl. Add vanilla extract, applesauce and honey. Add baking powder and almond meal. Mix till combined well.

2. Spray pan with non-stick spray. Heat on low. Once it's heated, add 3 tbsp. +/- of the batter.

3. Allow batter to cook for three to four minutes on first side, till it is firm enough to be flipped.

4. Cook second side for about two to three minutes, till cooked fully. Repeat this with other pancakes.

5. Serve with syrup.

Spiced Carrots & Cauliflower

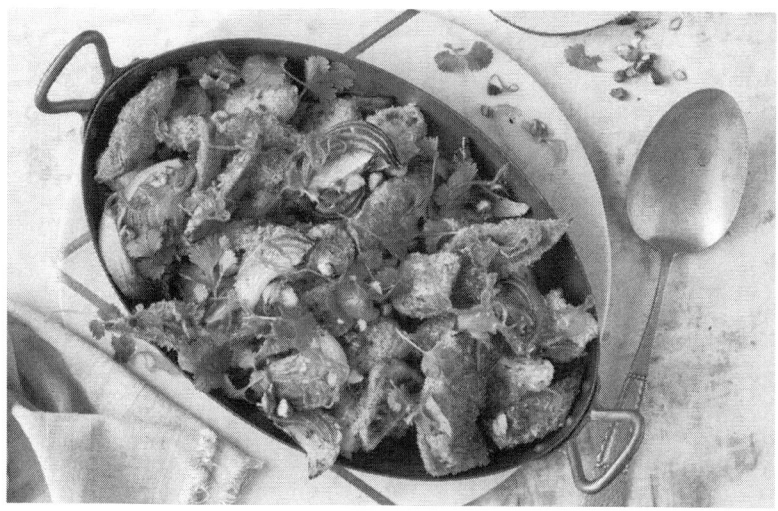

Here is a wonderful Indian recipe for a side dish that is sure to be a hit. You will sauté peas, cauliflower and carrots and add roasted ginger and cumin seeds for a tender, tasty dish.

Serves: 2

Time: 55 minutes

Ingredients:

- 2 tsp. of oil, olive
- 1 tsp. of cumin seeds
- 2 to 3 tbsp. of ginger, grated or chopped finely

- 1 chopped chili, green
- 1/2 tsp. of salt, sea
- 1/2 tsp. of turmeric
- 1/2 head of floret-chopped cauliflower
- 3/4 cup of carrots, chopped
- 1/2 cup of peas

Directions:

1. Heat oil to med-high in large sized pan.

2. Add the cumin seeds. Roast till they are fragrant, then reduce the heat to med.

3. Add chili and ginger. Cook for two to three minutes, till chili turns golden.

4. Add carrots and cauliflower. Cover pan and cook for four to five minutes.

5. Add the turmeric, peas and salt. Combine thoroughly. Reduce the heat down to low.

6. Cover. Cook till cauliflower becomes tender, or about 15-20 minutes. Top with cilantro and serve.

No-Grain Chilaquiles

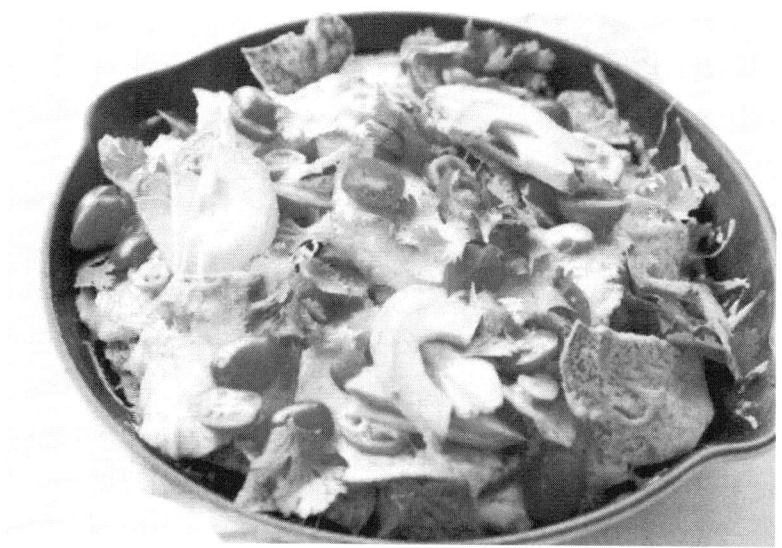

This recipe can be made with green or red enchilada sauce. The chilaquiles are great with plantain or taro chips, but any grain free chips will work fine.

Serves: 6

Time: 50 minutes

Ingredients:

- 1 tbsp. of butter, unsalted
- 6 eggs, large
- 1/2 tsp. of salt, sea

- Red enchilada sauce, bottled
- 12 oz. of plantain chips or other grain-free type
- 2 cups of cheese shreds, Monterey Jack
- 1/4 cup of jalapeños, pickled
- 2 sliced avocados
- 1/4 cup of salsa, mild or hot
- 1/4 cup of cilantro

Directions:

1. Preheat the oven to 400F.

2. Add the butter to oven-safe, large-sized skillet. Melt butter on med. heat.

3. Beat eggs. Pour into skillet. Stir occasionally while cooking till eggs are scrambled.

4. Season eggs with salt and spoon them into a small bowl. Set them aside.

5. Place 1/2 of plantain chips in skillet. Pour sauce (if using) over them. Toss till they are heated.

6. Place eggs and 1/2 of cheese atop chip mixture. Add the rest of the chips on the top.

7. Add jalapenos and remaining cheese. Place in oven. Bake for 8-10 minutes, to melt the cheese. Garnish with the salsa, avocados and cilantro. Serve.

Red Lentil Soup

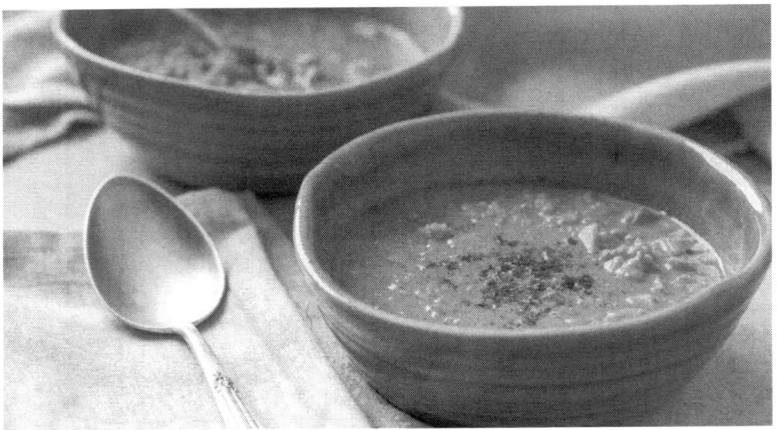

These Dals can be made with more or less water, for a thinner or thicker consistency. The chili and garlic make it authentically tasty. If you use less water for a thicker soup, it offers more lentils per serving, and thus more protein.

Serves: 2

Time: 1 hour & 25 minutes

Ingredients:

For lentils:

- 1/2 cup of dry orange/red/pink lentils
- 1 & 1/2 to 2 cups of water to mix

- 1/4 tsp. of turmeric
- 1/3 to 1/2 tsp. of salt, sea

For tempering:

- 2 tsp. of oil, olive
- 1/2 tsp. of cumin seeds
- 1/2 chopped pepper, serrano chili, as desired
- 3 sliced garlic cloves
- 3 to 4 tbsp. of red onion, chopped
- 1 generous dash curry powder

Directions:

1. To prepare lentils, wash them and then drain well.

2. Add them to a deep pan with 1 & 1/2 cups of filtered water, then turmeric and salt, as desired. Cover pan partially and cook at med-low till they are tender. This usually takes about 20 minutes.

3. For tempering, add oil to small pan on med. heat. Add cumin seeds. Cook for several seconds till they become fragrant and change color.

4. Add chili and garlic. Cook till garlic becomes golden brown in color. Add onion and cook till it is translucent.

5. Add dash of curry powder and combine. Taste. Adjust seasoning as desired. Serve while hot.

Crème Fraiche Carrots & Apricots

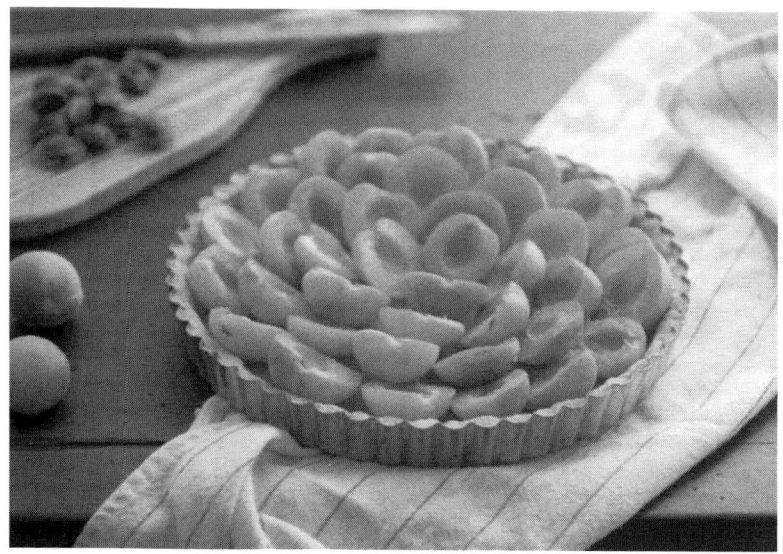

In this recipe, carrots are cooked with butter and seasoned with salt, and you can plump the dried fruits in liquor or juice if you like, to increase the flavor. The salty, sweet creaminess **Serves:** a wonderful combination.

Serves: 4

Time: 1/2 hour

Ingredients:

For carrots:

- 1 lb. of peeled, halved lengthways carrots
- 2 tbsp. of butter, unsalted
- 1/2 tsp. of salt, sea

For apricots:

- 1/4 cup of orange juice, fresh
- 1/4 cup of apricots, chopped and dried

For toppings:

- 1/2 cup of crème fraiche
- 1/4 cup of hazelnuts, chopped
- 1/4 cup of chopped parsley, flat-leaf type
- 1 tbsp. of honey, raw

Directions:

1. Melt butter on med. heat in large sized skillet.

2. Place carrots in a single layer. Cook for four to five minutes till edges start to turn brown.

3. Flip with tongs and continue to cook until other side also turns golden brown.

4. Place apricots and orange juice in small size saucepan. Bring to simmer on low heat, then remove from heat. Drain.

5. Spread crème fraiche on platter. Top with the apricots, parsley, hazelnuts and carrots. Drizzle over the top with honey and serve promptly.

Creamy Tomato Soup

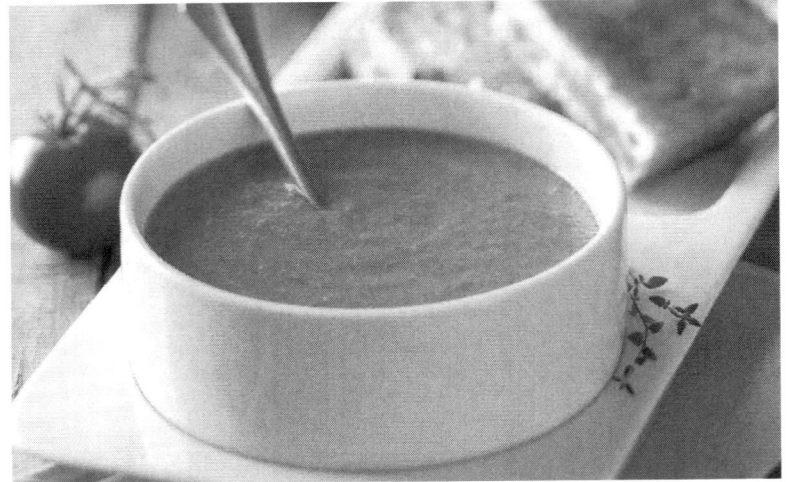

This is like cream of tomato soup, but without any cream. The recipe is an easy one– just blend it and go– it offers flavor, nutrient-richness and whole food goodness.

Serves: 4

Time: 10 minutes

Ingredients:

- 4 tomatoes, Roma
- 1/2 cup of tomatoes, sun-dried
- 1/2 cup of macadamia nuts, raw
- 1 tsp. of salt, sea

- 1/4 cup of basil, fresh
- 1/2 tsp. of pepper, white
- 1/4 tsp. of pepper, black
- 1 garlic clove
- 4 cups of water, hot

Directions:

1. Add all the ingredients to high-powered blender.

2. Blend on the high setting for five minutes, till the mixture is heated completely through.

3. Serve.

Shrimp Ceviche

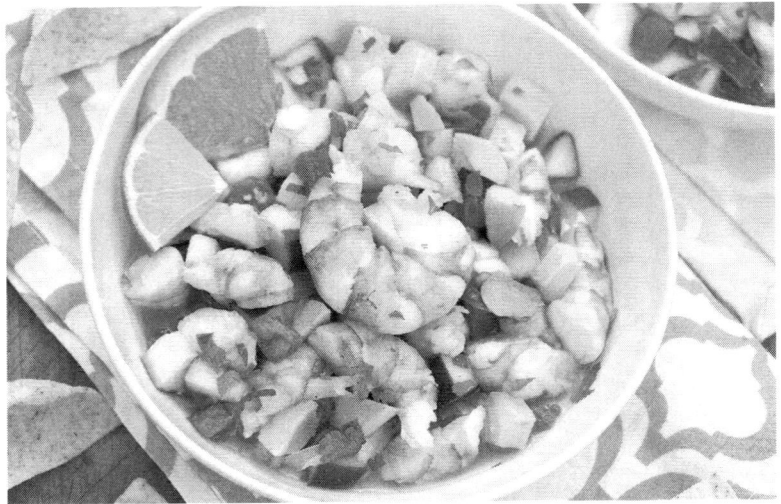

Ceviche is made with shellfish or raw fish, along with lime juice, onions, tomatoes and cilantro. The lime juice "cooks" the fish and the end result, after it is tossed with the remainder of the ingredients, is very refreshing.

Serves: 6-8

Time: 50 minutes

Ingredients:

- 1 lb. of peeled, cubed shrimp, wild, raw
- 1/2 cup of lime juice, fresh

- 1 pint of halved tomatoes, cherry
- 1/2 cup chopped each of red onion, cucumber and cilantro leaves, fresh
- 1 de-veined, de-seeded, chopped jalapeno pepper
- 1/2 tsp. of salt, sea

Directions:

1. Place the lime juice and shrimp in shallow, medium dish. Cover it and place in refrigerator for 1/2 hour, to marinate.

2. Place the shrimp/lime mixture, sea salt, jalapeno pepper, cilantro, red onion and tomatoes in medium sized bowl.

3. Stir till incorporated well. Season as desired and serve cold.

Slow-Cooker Pork

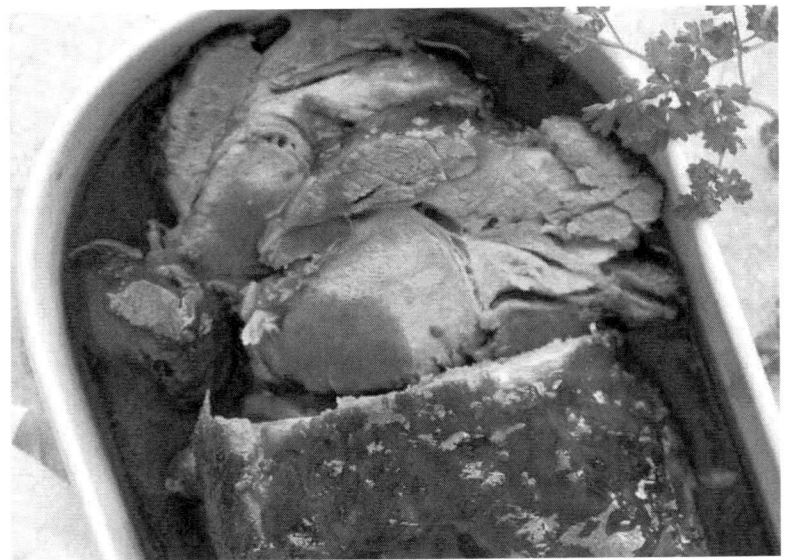

This recipe can be made with slow cooked pork or beef. It is added to ginger root beer, sweetened with Stevia, along with a BBQ sauce sweetened with honey. It's SO tasty!

Serves: 6

Time: 10 minutes + 9 hours slow cooker time

Ingredients:

- 1 & 3/4 pounds of shoulder roast, pork
- 1/2 tsp. of paprika

- 1/4 tsp. of garlic powder
- 1/4 tsp. of onion powder
- 3/4 can of root beer, sugar-free, sweetened with Stevia
- 1/2 cup of BBQ sauce, sugar-free, sweetened with honey

Directions:

1. Remove twine from shoulder roast. Place in slow cooker. Sprinkle with onion and garlic powders and paprika.

2. Pour root beer alongside of pork.

3. Cover. Cook on low heat for nine hours in slow cooker.

4. Drain juices. Return meat to slow cooker. Shred the meat using a fork.

5. Add BBQ sauce and stir. Cook on the low setting for one more hour.

6. Serve with veggies.

Herbed Braised Beans

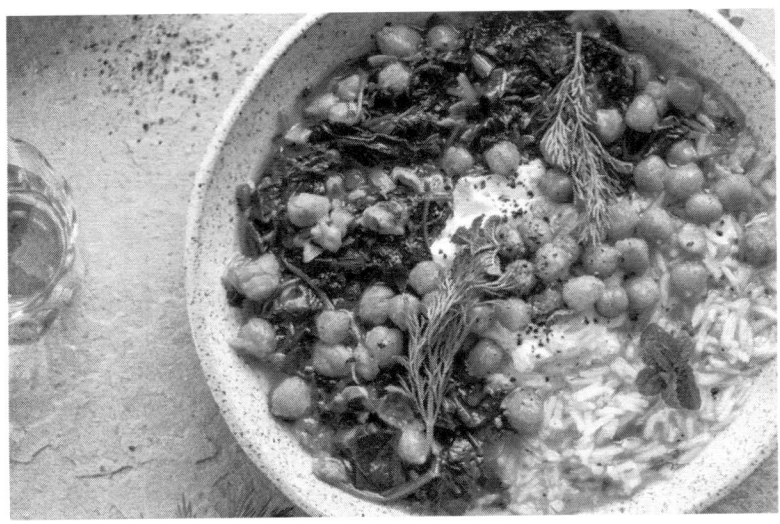

Braised beans make an incredible comfort food, especially in the colder months of winter. They store well as leftovers, too.

Serves: 8

Time: 4 hours & 25 minutes + 8 hours soaking time for beans

Ingredients:

- 1 cup of white navy or cannellini beans– soak overnight

- 1 cup of chickpeas, dried – soak overnight
- 2 tbsp. of butter, unsalted
- 1 chopped onion
- 3 chopped garlic cloves
- 2 chopped celery stalks
- 1 x 24-oz. jar of tomatoes, crushed
- 4 cups of stock, chicken
- 3 sprigs of rosemary, fresh
- 3 sprigs of thyme, fresh
- 1 head of chopped kale
- 2 tsp. of salt, sea
- 1/2 tsp. of black pepper, fresh ground

Directions:

1. Place beans and chickpeas in large sized bowl. Cover with filtered water. Add a couple pinches baking soda. Allow to soak at room temp overnight.

2. Next day, drain and rinse the beans. Melt the butter in large sized pot on med. heat. Add celery, onion and garlic. Cook for four to five minutes, till barely tender.

3. Add tomatoes, thyme, rosemary, beans and stock. Bring to boil.

4. Reduce heat to simmer. Allow to cook till beans become tender, or about four hours.

15-20 minutes before you serve, bring pot of salted water to boil. Add kale. Cook for eight minutes. Drain.

5. When beans become tender, add and stir cooked kale, salt and ground pepper.

6. Serve.

Lemon-Kissed Bean Salad

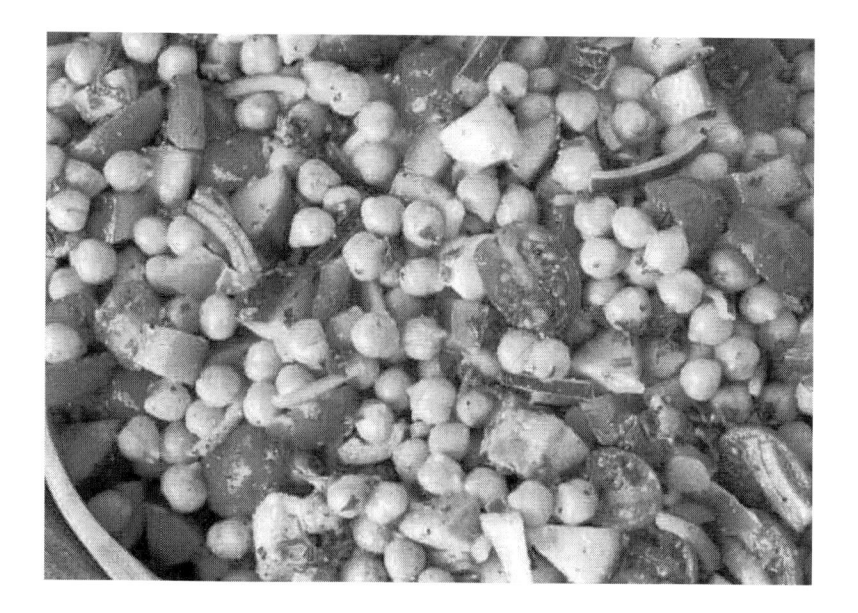

This Lemon-Kissed bean salad is packed with protein and filled with zesty, refreshing colors and flavors. It serves a great side dish or healthy lunch.

Serves: 6

Time: 20 minutes

Ingredients:

- 1 x 14-oz. can of chickpeas or cannellini beans
- 6 oz. of trimmed, 1-inch cut green beans

- 1/4 cup of tender-stemmed parsley leaves, fresh,
- 1/4 cup of oil, olive
- 3 tbsp. of chives, chopped
- 2 tbsp. of capers, chopped
- 1 tbsp. of lemon zest, finely grated
- 2 tbsp. of lemon juice, fresh
- 1/2 tsp. of pepper, Aleppo
- Salt, sea
- Pepper, black ground

Directions:

1. Toss rinsed chickpeas or cannellini beans with 6 oz. of green beans, parsley leaves, olive oil, fresh chives, lemon zest, capers, Aleppo pepper and lemon juice in large sized bowl.

2. Season using sea salt and ground pepper.

3. Serve.

Mango Chicken Salad

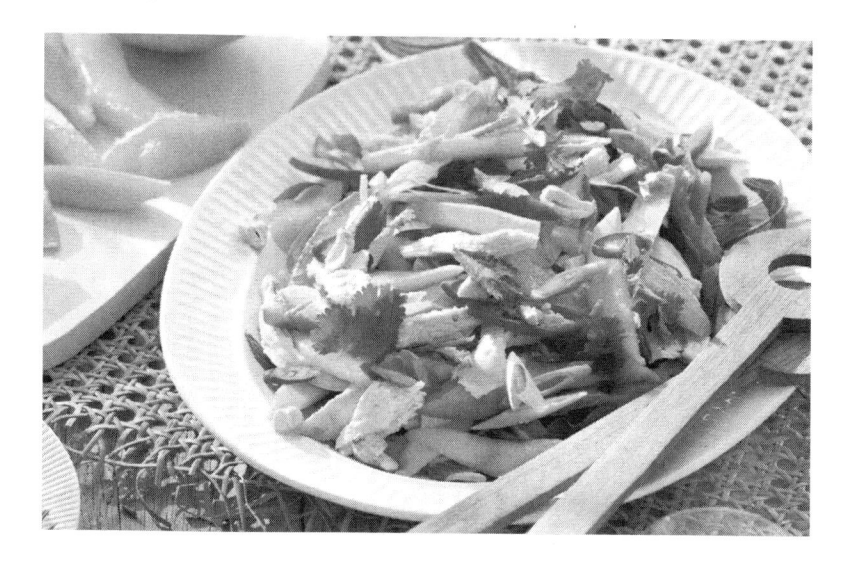

Chicken salad with herbs and fruits is among my favorite dishes to eat in the summertime. It goes well with other salads, to make a light meal, or spooned into lettuce wraps for a quick meal.

Serves: 4-6

Time: 20 minutes

Ingredients:

For dressing:

- 3 tbsp. of lime juice, fresh

- 1 shallot
- 2 tbsp. of fish sauce
- 1 clove of garlic
- 1 pinch pepper flakes, red
- 1/2 tsp. of honey, raw
- 1/2 tsp. of oil, sesame

For chicken:

- 4 cups chicken, shredded, cooked
- For salad:
- 2 peeled, pitted, cubed mangos
- 1/2 cup each of chopped mint, fresh; chopped cilantro and chopped basil

Directions:

1. Place dressing ingredients in food processor. Blend till texture is smooth.

2. Place chicken, mango, basil, mint and cilantro in medium sized bowl. Pour the dressing over it.

3. Toss and coat well. Serve.

Broccoli & Roast Salmon

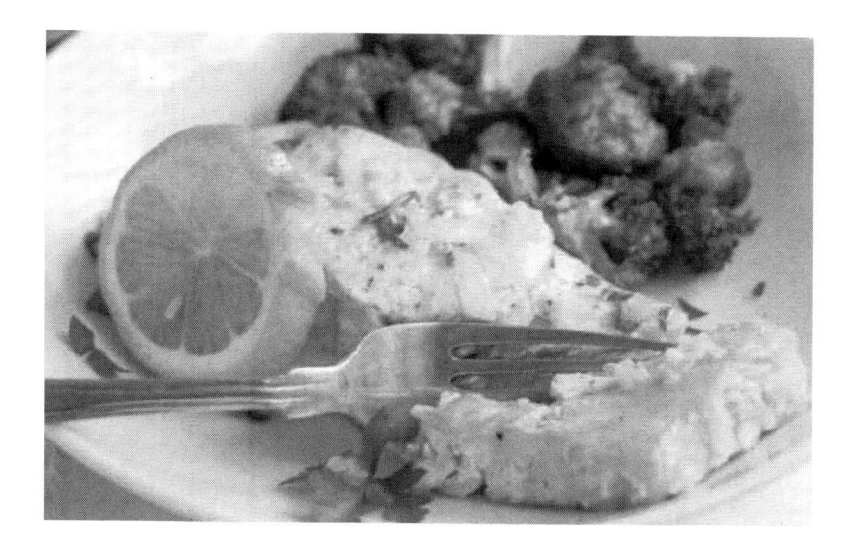

When you give the broccoli time to brown before you prepare the salmon, it coaxes out the natural sweetness. This is an easy to make and tasty dish for any lunch or dinner.

Serves: 4

Time: 50 minutes

Ingredients:

- 1 floret-sliced bunch of broccolis
- 4 tbsp. of oil, olive
- Salt, kosher

- Pepper, fresh ground
- 4 x 6-oz. salmon fillets, skinless
- 1 ring-sliced jalapeno pepper
- 2 tbsp. of vinegar, rice, unseasoned
- 2 tbsp. of capers, drained

Directions:

1. Preheat the oven to 400F.

2. Toss 2 tbsp. of oil and broccoli on rimmed cookie sheet. Season with kosher salt and ground pepper.

3. Roast the broccoli and toss it occasionally, till tender but crisp. This usually takes about 12 to 15 minutes.

4. Rub the salmon with 1 tbsp. of oil. Season as desired.

5. Push the broccoli out to edge of baking sheet. Put salmon in middle. Roast till the salmon is opaque all over and the broccoli becomes tender. This will typically take 10 to 15 minutes.

6. Combine vinegar, jalapeno and 1 pinch salt in a small sized bowl. Allow it to sit till the jalapeno has softened

slightly. Mix in the capers and the last 1 tbsp. of oil. Season as desired.

7. Drizzle vinaigrette over broccoli and salmon. Serve.

Shrimp with Grits

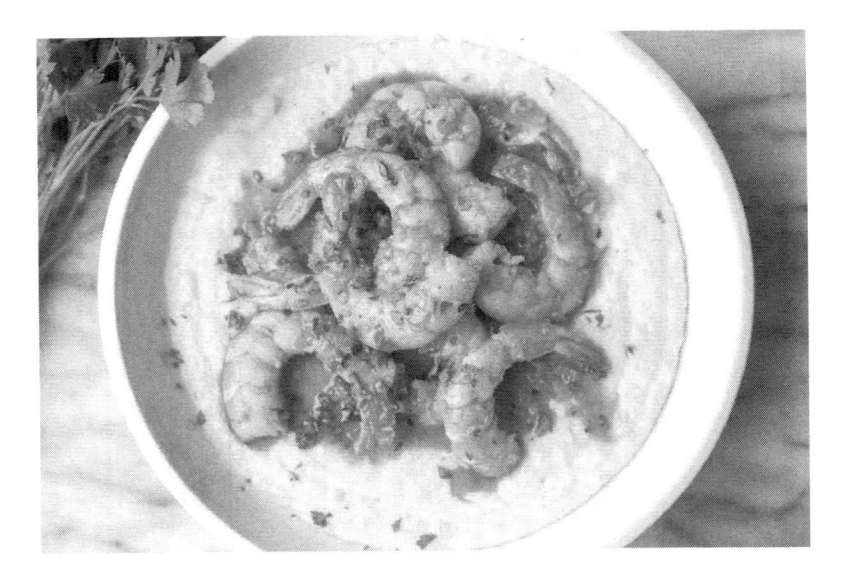

This recipe contains corn, and this grain-free recipe is much healthier, with almost the same taste.

Serves: 4

Time: 45 minutes

Ingredients:

For grits:

- 4 tbsp. of butter, unsalted
- 1 head of riced cauliflower

- 1/2 cup of chopped onions
- 3 chopped garlic heads
- 1/2 tsp. of salt, sea
- 2 tbsp. of cream, raw

For shrimp with sauce:

- 2 tbsp. of butter, unsalted
- 1/2 cup of onions, chopped
- 8 oz. of chopped mushrooms
- 2 cups of spinach
- 1 cup of broth, chicken
- 2 tbsp. of cream, heavy
- 1 lb. of peeled, de-veined shrimp, wild
- 1/2 tsp. of seasoning salt
- 1/4 tsp. of paprika
- 1/2 tsp. of garlic powder

Directions:

1. Melt butter on med. heat in large sized skillet. Add sea salt, garlic, onions and cauliflower. Sauté for 8-10 minutes till cauliflower softens.

2. Pour cauliflower mixture in food processor. Add cream. Pulse 10 x 1-second till mixture matches grits in consistency.

3. Wipe skillet that you used for grits. Melt 2 tbsp. of butter in that skillet on med. heat.

4. Add mushrooms and onions. Cook for eight to 10 minutes, till they soften and begin turning brown around edges.

5. Add spinach. Cook till it wilts. Add cream and broth. Simmer till sauce has been reduced by 1/2 and starts thickening.

6. Toss shrimp, seasoning mix, garlic powder and paprika in small sized bowl. Add seasoned shrimp to mushroom sauce. Stir occasionally as you cook for five to seven minutes, till shrimp cooks through.

7. Spoon some grits in bowls. Top with mushroom and shrimp sauce. Serve.

Chili Gremolata Roasted Shrimp

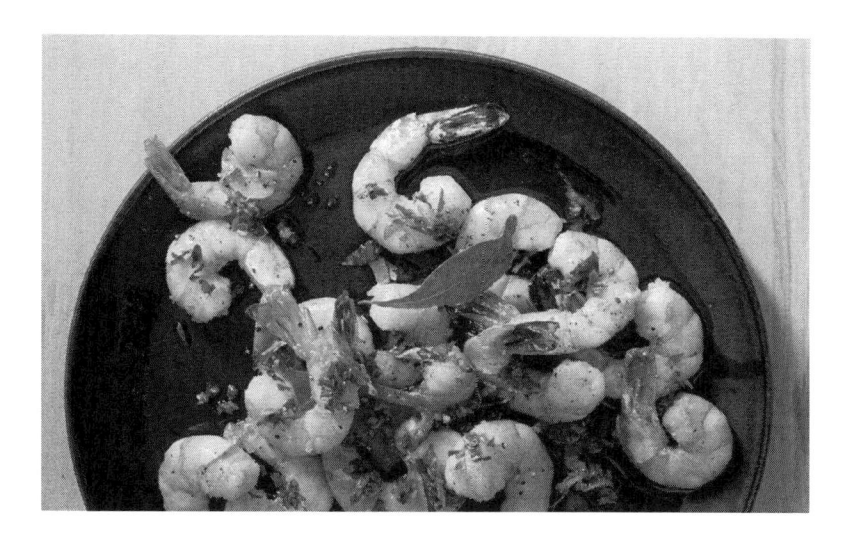

This is a wonderful dish that I like to serve with grain-free alternatives to bread or rice, so we can sop up the wonderful cooking liquid and its intense flavor.

Serves: 4

Time: 20 minutes

Ingredients:

For the shrimp:

- 2 halved lengthways red serrano chilies
- 6 sliced cloves of garlic

- 2 bay leaves, dried
- 1/2 cup of oil, olive
- 1 & 1/2 lbs. peeled and de-veined shrimp, large
- 1 wedge-cut lemon

For Chili Gremolata (herb condiment) and the assembly:

- 1 de-seeded, chopped serrano chili, red
- 1 grated clove of garlic
- chopped cilantro and parsley, fresh, 1/4 cup each
- 1 tbsp. of lemon zest, grated finely
- 1 tbsp. of oil, olive
- Salt, kosher
- Pepper, fresh ground

Directions:

1. Preheat the oven to 450F. Heat the bay leaves, oil, garlic and chilies in small sized saucepan on med.

2. Heat till the mixture begins sizzling. Remove from heat.

3. Toss the shrimp and chili oil in medium baking dish. Roast and turn when it is halfway done, till the shrimp cook through, about eight to 10 minutes.

4. For gremolata, mix the chili, oil, zest, herbs and garlic in small sized bowl. Season as desired.

5. Squeeze fresh lemon on shrimp and top them with gremolata. Serve.

Steak Vinaigrette with Vegetables

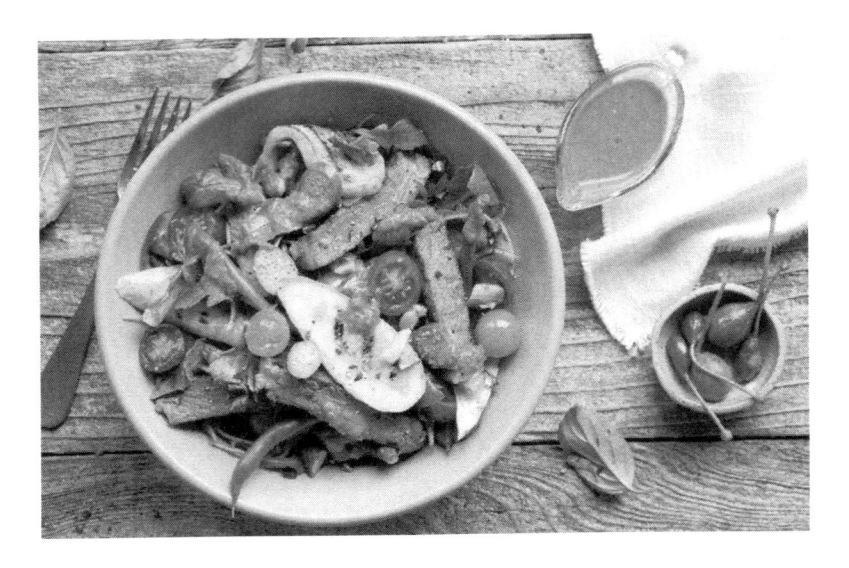

This meal is so tasty that my family often craves it again the next day! So, I often make a double recipe. It is satisfying, refreshing and a great summertime dish.

Serves: 4

Time: 45 minutes

Ingredients:

For veggies:

- 1 lb. of washed, trimmed green beans
- 2 pints of tomatoes, grape or cherry

- 1 tbsp. of clarified butter, melted
- 1/4 tsp. of salt, sea

For steaks:

- 3 steaks– skirt, sirloin or ribeye
- Salt, sea

For vinaigrette:

- 1 shallot
- 3 tbsp. of vinegar, red wine
- 1 garlic clove
- 6 tbsp. of oil, olive
- 1 cup of basil, fresh
- 1/4 tsp. of salt, sea

Directions:

1. Preheat oven to 425F.

2. Place tomatoes and green beans in large sized baking dish. Add sea salt and clarified butter. Combine by tossing.

3. Roast the vegetables for 18-20 minutes, till tomato skins start bursting and green beans become golden around edges.

4. Preheat grill on med-high. Season both sides of steaks with salt. Grill for 2-3 minutes per side until done as you desire. Place steaks on plate. Allow to rest for 8-10 minutes.

5. Place oil, sea salt, basil, vinegar, garlic and shallot in blender. Blend till you have a smooth texture.

6. Cut steaks into strips against grain. Serve with the veggies, drizzled with basil vinaigrette.

Southwestern Style Squash Soup

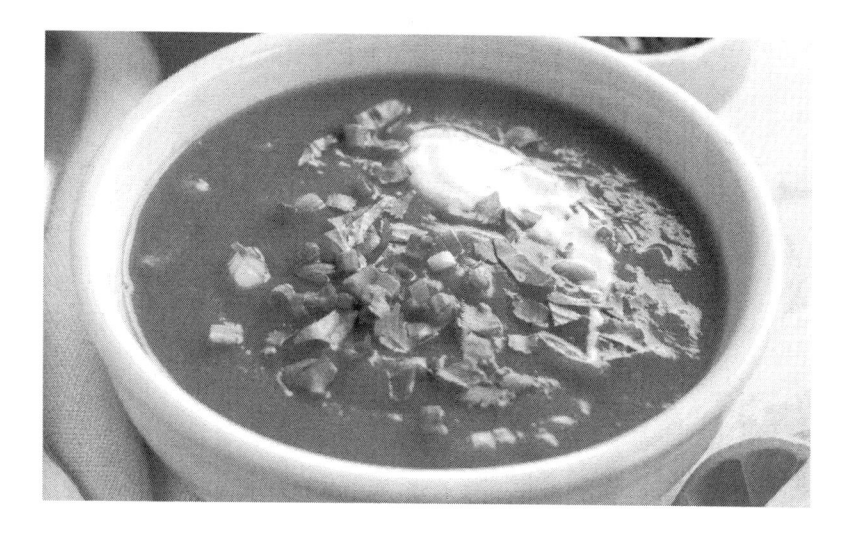

This soup is hearty and robust, and you can even make a meal from it. It's filled with protein and fiber and tastes so great that everyone wants seconds.

Serves: 3-4

Time: 1 hour 40 minutes

Ingredients:

- 1 squash, medium
- 1 tbsp. of oil, canola
- 1 diced onion, small
- 2 stalks of diced celery

- 2 cloves of crushed garlic
- 2 tsp. of cumin
- Ground chilies, as desired
- 1/2 tsp. of pepper, ground
- 1/4 tsp. of salt, kosher
- 4 cups of stock, vegetable
- 1 cup of cauliflower rice, prepared
- 1 cup of black beans

To garnish:

- Cilantro, chopped
- Green onion, chopped
- Avocado, diced

Directions:

1. Slice squash in half. Scoop out the seeds. Then roast it in 350F oven for 40-45 minutes, till it becomes soft. Scoop out flesh. Set aside.

2. Chop vegetables. Fry onion in pan with canola oil. Add salt, ground pepper, chili, cumin and garlic after the onion sweats.

3. Puree squash in food processor with all frying pan ingredients.

4. Combine this mixture with vegetable stock in pot. Bring to simmer.

5. Once mixture simmers, add beans and cauliflower rice.

6. Simmer for 10 or more minutes, so the flavors can mingle. Squash will thicken up its consistency.

7. Season as desired. Top with your desired garnishes. Serve.

Lemon Chicken with Veggies

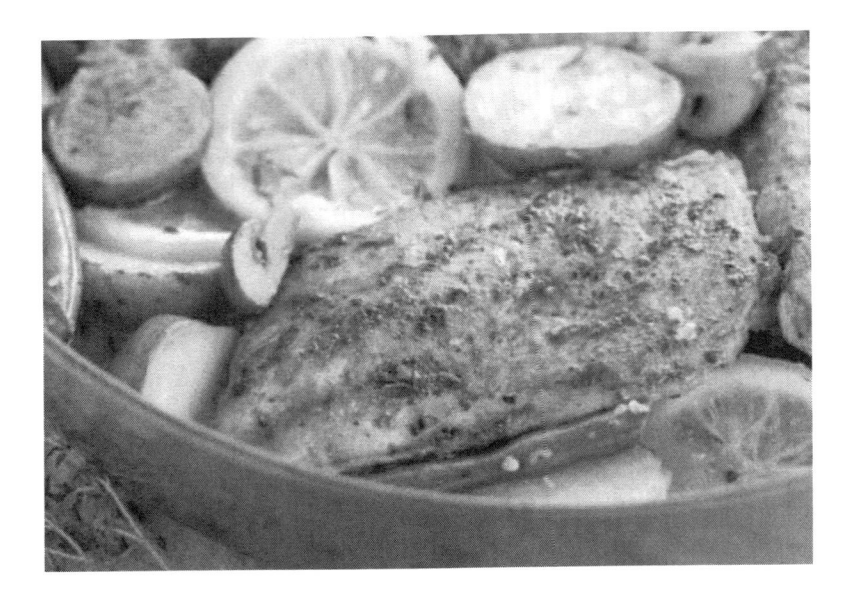

This is a wonderful chicken recipe. It's also easy to make, and it's packed with flavor. The artichoke hearts and spinach give it a special taste.

Serves: 4

Time: 45 minutes

Ingredients:

- 1 & 1/4 cups of stock, chicken
- 4 oz. of cream cheese
- 1 tbsp. of flour, arrowroot

- 1/2 tsp. of salt, sea
- 4 chicken breasts, skinless, boneless
- Salt, sea, and ground pepper to season
- 1/2 cup of flour, almond
- 2 tbsp. of butter
- 2 tbsp. of oil, olive
- 4 chopped garlic cloves
- 1 tbsp. of thyme, fresh
- 12 oz. of spinach, baby
- 1 pkg. of frozen & thawed, chopped artichoke hearts
- 1 fresh lemon, juice only

Directions:

1. Place salt, arrow root flour, cream cheese and stock in food processor. Blend till combined well. Set it aside.

2. Season chicken as desired. Dredge in the almond flour and shake off excess.

3. Heat large sized cast iron skillet on med. heat for two minutes. Add 1 tbsp. of oil and butter. Swirl and coat pan.

4. Add chicken in one layer. Cook and flip once, till chicken is cooked through and golden brown. Transfer to plate.

5. Add garlic, thyme and remaining oil to empty skillet. Cook till mixture is fragrant, which will only take 15-20 seconds.

6. Add spinach. Stir frequently while cooking till spinach wilts. Add and stir artichokes.

7. Add chicken stock mixture. Stir constantly while cooking till sauce starts thickening.

8. Return chicken and juices to pan. Remove pan from heat.

9. Spritz lemon juice on top. Serve with cauliflower rice.

Kelp Noodles with Sesame

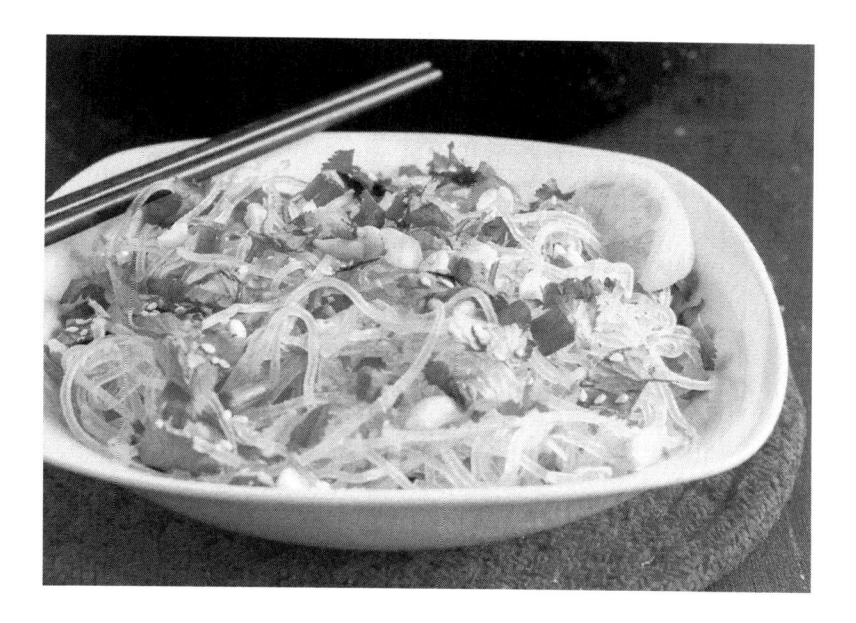

Once you enjoy this gluten free sesame noodle recipe once, you'll be hooked. It's every bit as good as the traditional dish. This recipe uses kelp noodles, which are low in carbs, too.

Serves: 2

Time: 50 minutes

Ingredients:

- 1 pkg. of noodles, kelp
- 1/4 cup of almond butter, roasted, creamy
- 1 tbsp. of sesame oil, toasted
- 2 to 3 tsp. of vinegar, Ume Plum
- 3 drops of Stevia sweetener

Directions:

1. To soften the noodles, rinse through a strainer. Place the noodles in medium sized bowl and fill it with lemon juice and warm salted water. Allow to sit for 1/2 hour, then rinse the noodles and strain them.

2. In small sized bowl, combine Stevia, vinegar, sesame oil and almond butter. 3. Toss the noodles with the sauce created in step.

3. Serve.

Ham & White Bean Slow Cooker Soup

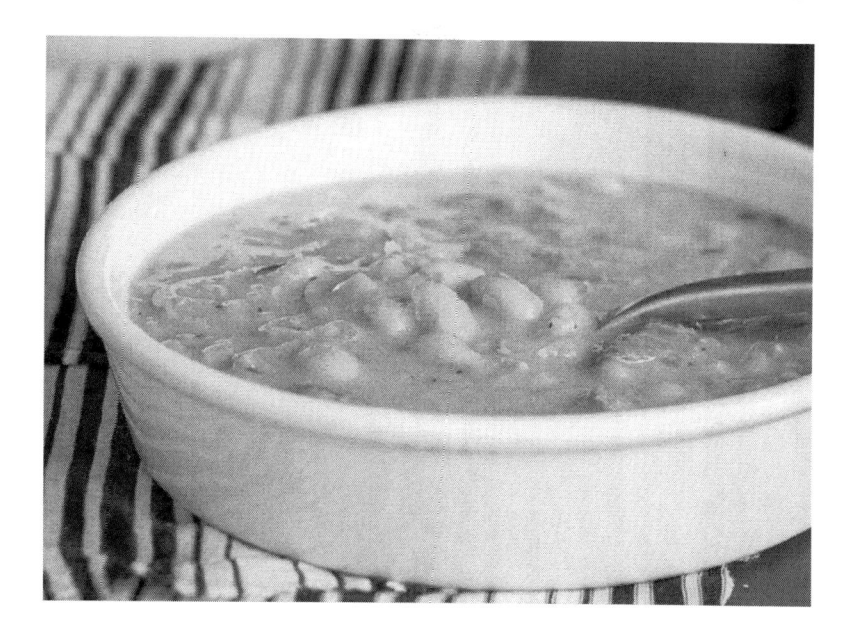

Nourishing soups make the cooler months of the year easier to deal with. This soup is comforting and warm, and a slow cooker does most of the work for you.

Serves: 6-8

Time: 10 minutes + 6 hours slow cooker time + 8 hours for bean soaking

Ingredients:

For beans:

- 1 lb. of navy beans, white, dried – soaked overnight
- Baking soda– a pinch

For soup:

- 2 ham hocks, smoked, meaty
- 8 cups of stock, chicken
- 6 cubed celery ribs
- 6 round-cut carrots
- 1 chopped onion, yellow
- 10 peeled, smashed garlic cloves
- 6 sprigs of thyme, fresh
- 2 tsp. of salt, sea

Directions:

1. On the night before cooking, place beans in large sized bowl. Cover with filtered water. Add pinch of baking soda and stir. Allow to sit overnight.

2. Next day, pour beans from bowl and drain and rinse them. Place in slow cooker. Add thyme, garlic, onion, carrots,

celery, stock and ham hocks. Combine by stirring. Cover. Cook on low for about 6 hours or so, till beans become tender.

3. Remove ham hocks and thyme with tongs. Shred ham. Return meat to slow cooker. Season as desired. Serve hot.

Asian Vegetable Stir Fry

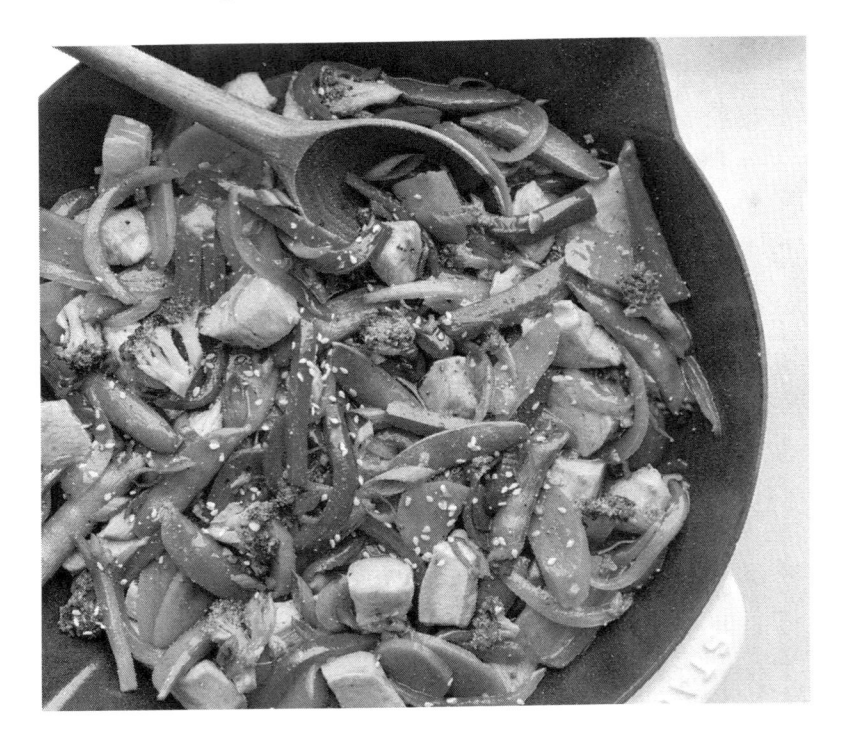

This Paleo-friendly dish is a healthy entrée for a grain-free eater, too. The combination is so tempting, with its chicken, cauliflower rice and veggies sautéed in tasty coconut oil.

Serves: 4

Time: 1 & 1/4 hours

Ingredients:

- 1 lb. of chicken breast, skinless, boneless
- 2 tbsp. of oil, coconut
- 1 chopped onion, medium
- 2 spear-sliced broccoli heads
- 2 sliced carrots, medium
- 2 sliced in strips heads of baby Bok choy
- 4 oz. of de-stemmed, sliced mushrooms, shiitake
- 1 sliced zucchini, small
- 1/2 tsp. of salt, sea
- 1 & 1/2 cups of water, filtered
- 2 tbsp. of arrow root powder
- 2 tbsp. of sesame oil, toasted
- 2 tbsp. of vinegar, plum

Directions:

1. Rinse chicken. Pat it dry.

2. Cut in 1" cubes. Transfer them to plate.

3. Heat coconut oil on med. heat.

4. Sauté onion for eight to 10 minutes, till translucent and soft.

5. Add chicken, broccoli and carrots. Sauté for eight to 10 minutes, till nearly tender.

6. Add sea salt, zucchini, mushrooms and Bok choy. Sauté for three to five minutes.

7. Add a cup of filtered water. Cover fry pan. Cook for 10 minutes, till veggies wilt.

8. Dissolve arrow root powder in small bowl with 1/2 cup water. Stir till they are combined well.

9. Add arrow root mixture to veggies. Cook, while stirring, for three minutes, till sauce becomes glossy and thickens.

10. Add vinegar and sesame oil. Stir. Serve.

Grain-Free Potatoes & Roast Chicken

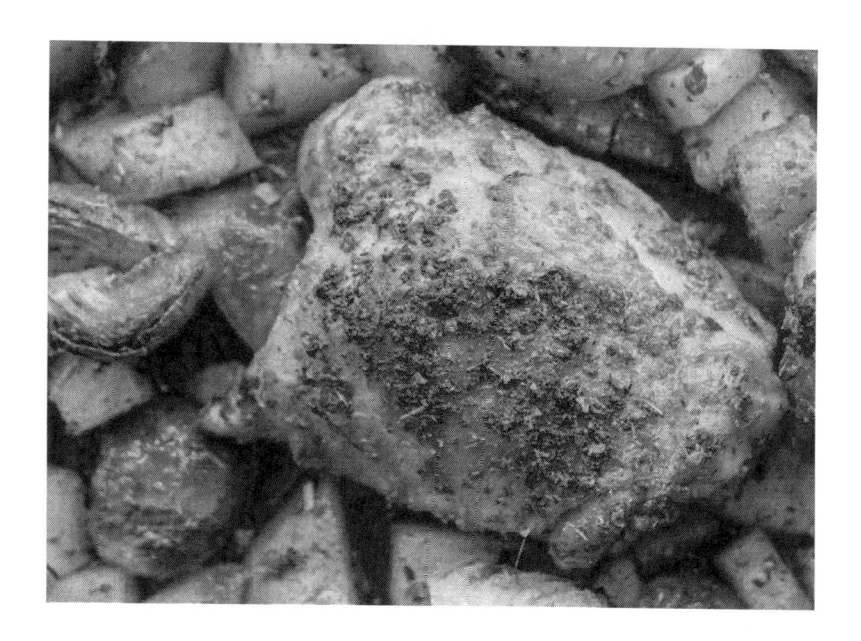

Most families enjoy chicken and potatoes, and mine is no exception. You can make it with potatoes and serve with another veggie or a salad. Potatoes can work in the place of other veggies, too.

Serves: 6

Time: 1 1/2 hours

Ingredients:

- 1 whole chicken, organic

- 2 tbsp. of melted, clarified butter
- 6 thinly-sliced potatoes, medium
- Sea salt & black, ground pepper

Directions:

1. Preheat oven to 425F.

2. Place chicken in large oven-safe skillet. Brush 1 tbsp. of clarified butter over it.

3. Place potatoes in large sized bowl. Toss with the rest of clarified butter. Pour buttery potatoes into skillet, around chicken. Season as desired.

4. Roast chicken and potatoes for 40-45 minutes, till chicken skin is golden and thermometer inserted in chicken shows 165F.

5. Transfer chicken carefully to work surface. Place potatoes in skillet back in oven.

6. Tent chicken with aluminum foil. Allow to set for 18-20 minutes. Potatoes should be left in to continue roasting.

7. After 18-20 minutes, take potatoes from oven. Carve chicken. Serve.

Pumpkin Roll Cake

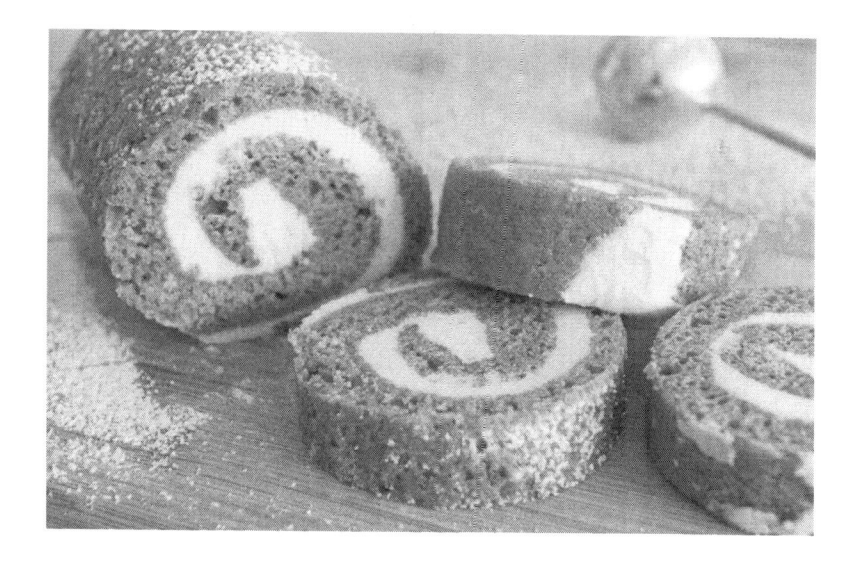

This roll cake is much easier to make than you would think. After the cake has cooled it will unroll quite easily, to be spread with cream cheese and rolled back up.

Serves: 8-10

Time: 50 minutes

Ingredients:

For cake:

- 3 eggs, large
- 1/2 cup of sugar, maple

- 2/3 cup of organic pumpkin, pureed
- 1/4 cup each of flour, coconut, tapioca and arrow root
- 1/2 tsp. of gluten-free baking powder
- 1/2 tsp. of baking soda
- 1 & 1/2 tbsp. of spice, pumpkin pie
- 1/8 tsp. of salt, sea

For filling:

- 1/2 cup of sugar, maple
- 2 tsp. of flour, arrow root
- 8 oz. of cream cheese, softened
- 2 tbsp. of butter, unsalted, softened
- 1 tsp. of vanilla extract, pure

Directions:

1. Preheat oven to 350F.

2. Oil or butter 18x13" baking sheet. Line with baking paper.

3. Place sugar and eggs in bowl of standing mixer with attached beater. Mix at med-high level for about eight minutes, till the mixture is thickened and a pale yellow in color. Fold in pumpkin.

4. Place sea salt, pumpkin pie spice, baking soda, baking powder, arrow root, tapioca and coconut flour in medium sized bowl. Combine by whisking. Remove clumps, if any. Fold flour mixture into egg mixture.

5. Pour batter onto baking sheet. Spread batter gently with spatula till it is even across pan.

6. Bake at 350F for 10-12 minutes. Remove from oven. Allow to sit for about five minutes.

7. Sprinkle cake with a bit of arrow root. Place large dish towel over entire cake. Put oven mitts on. Grasp ends of pan. Turn cake over onto dish towel.

8. Peel baking paper off carefully. Roll towel and cake up together. Allow to completely cool.

9. Place 2 tsp. of arrow root flour and 1/2 cup of maple sugar into coffee grinder. Grind till you have a fine powder.

10. Place vanilla extract, butter, sugar mixture and cream cheese in medium bowl. Beat with mixer till mixture is fluffy, or about two to three minutes.

11. Unroll cake carefully. Spread cream cheese over cake with spatula. Re-roll cake. Serve or cover and refrigerate before serving.

Grain-Free Honey Cake

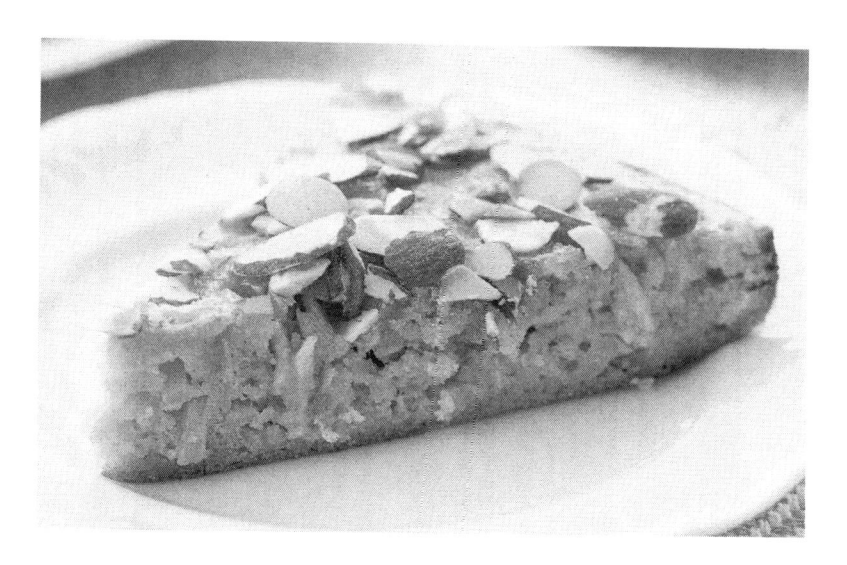

This is an easy, Paleo friendly recipe that you are bound to love. It's made with low-carb, healthy almond flour. It tastes amazingly like the original version but it's grain-free.

Serves: 12

Time: 1 hour & 25 minutes + 1 hour cooling time

Ingredients:

- 2 & 1/2 cups of almond flour, blanched
- 1/2 tsp. of salt, sea
- 1 tsp. of baking soda

- 1 tbsp. of cinnamon, ground
- 1/4 tsp. of cloves, ground
- 1/2 cup of honey, pure
- 1/4 cup of shortening, palm
- 4 eggs, large
- 1/2 cup of raisins

Directions:

1. Combine cloves, cinnamon, baking soda, salt and almond flour in large sized bowl.

2. Combine eggs, honey and shortening in separate bowl.

3. Combine wet ingredient mixture into dry mixture. Add raisins and stir.

4. Grease, then flour 8" spring form pan.

5. Set to bake at 350F oven for 30 to 35 minutes.

6. Remove from the oven. Cool for an hour. Serve.

Peach Cobbler

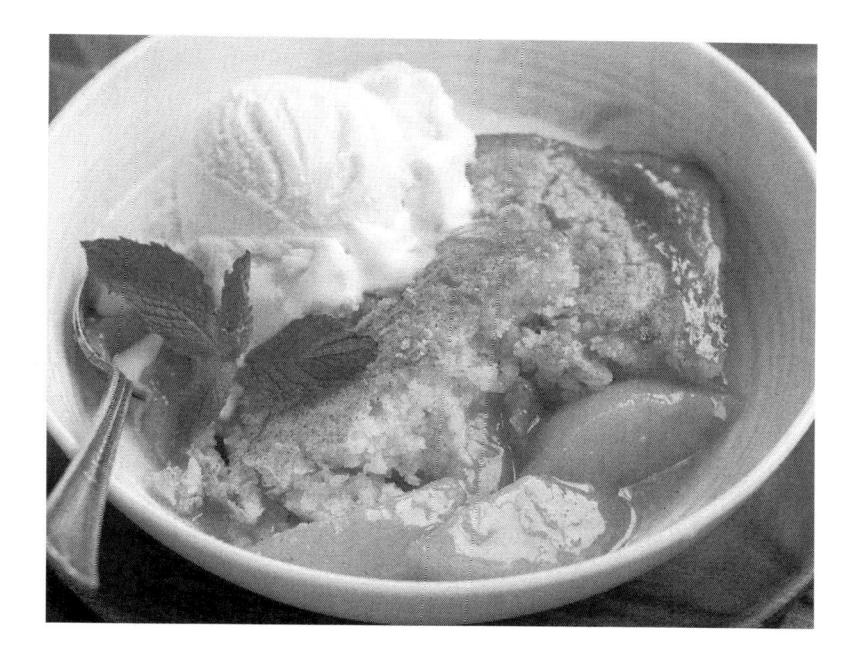

Everyone loves peach cobbler, it seems. Juicy, sweet peaches are topped with a buttery, fluffy topping that is a bit crisp, and it's a wonderful end to a healthy meal.

Serves: 6-8

Time: 1 hour & 20 minutes

Ingredients:

For peach filling:

- 10 cups of peeled, wedge-cut peaches, fresh
- 1/3 cup of sugar, maple
- 2 tbsp. of flour, arrow root
- 1 tbsp. of lemon juice, fresh
- 1/3 cup of water, filtered

For topping:

- 1/3 cup of each: tapioca, arrow root and coconut flours
- 1/4 tsp. of cinnamon, ground
- 1/2 cup + 1 tbsp. of sugar, maple
- 1 tsp. of baking powder
- 12 tbsp. of unsalted butter, cold
- 2 beaten eggs, large
- 1 tsp. of vanilla extract, pure

Directions:

1. Preheat oven to 350F.

2. Place peaches in large sized bowl. Remove 1/4 of peaches. Chop them up.

3. Combine chopped peaches, water, lemon juice, arrow root flour and maple sugar in medium sized saucepan. Heat on med. while stirring till liquid starts thickening.

4. Remove from heat. Pour hot peach mixture on remaining peaches. Stir and combine well. Pour peach mixture into 11x8" baking dish. Set it aside.

5. Place baking powder, 1/2 cup of sugar, cinnamon and flours in food processor. Pulse and combine. Add butter. Pulse 15 to 20 times till pea-sized.

6. Add vanilla and beaten eggs. Pulse till moistened evenly. Spoon dough dollops onto peaches. Sprinkle with last tbsp. of sugar.

7. Bake for 45-50 minutes till topping begins to turn golden brown.

8. Cool for 15-20 minutes before serving.

Apple-Cinnamon Grain-Free Cake

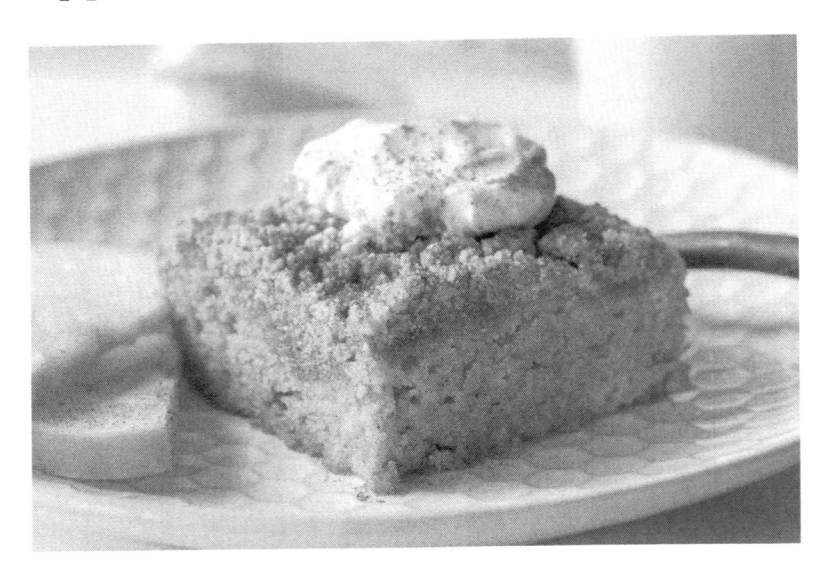

This is a special Autumn dessert and quite easily made. There are not many ingredients and even kids love it when smothered with whipped cream.

Serves: 12

Time: 50 minutes

Ingredients:

- 1 peeled, chopped, cored apple
- 2 tbsp. of freshly squeezed orange juice
- 1 cup of almond butter

- 1/4 cup of honey, pure
- 2 eggs, large
- 1 tbsp. of vanilla extract, pure
- 2 tbsp. cinnamon, ground
- 1/2 tsp. of salt, sea

Directions:

1. Pulse almond butter, apple and orange juice in food processor till blended well.

2. Pulse in cinnamon, salt, vanilla, eggs and honey.

3. Pour the batter into greased 8" square baking dish. 4. Bake in 350F oven for 30-35 minutes. Allow to cool, then serve.

Grain-Free Chocolate Cake

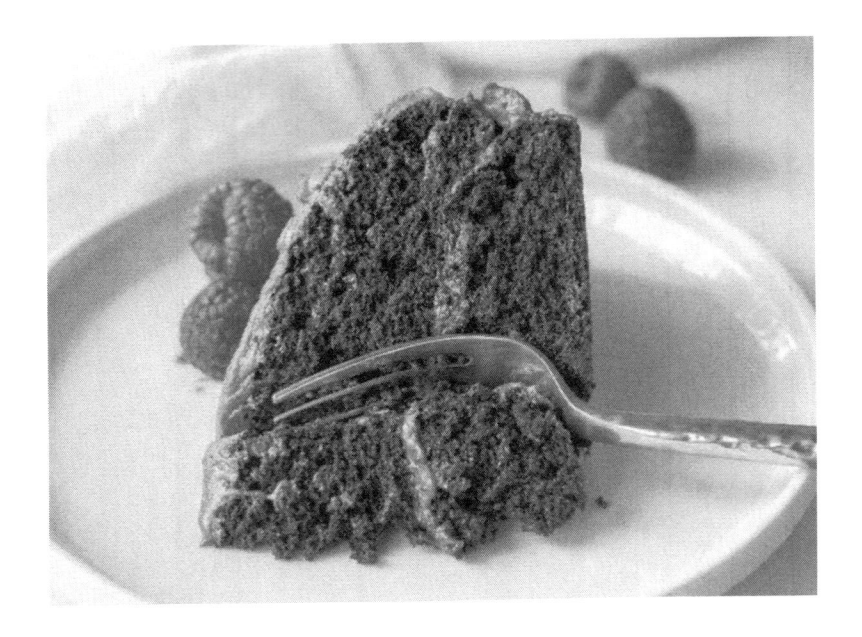

Celebrate a birthday– or any day– with this nut-free, dairy-free, grain-free chocolate cake. Everyone can enjoy it since it has only healthy ingredients.

Serves: 10-12

Time: 1 hour & 10 minutes

Ingredients:

For cake:

- 1 cup of flour, coconut
- 1/2 tsp. of salt, sea
- 1 tsp. of baking soda
- 8 oz. of melted chocolate, semi-sweet
- 1/2 cup of syrup, maple
- 8 eggs, large
- 1/2 cup of yogurt, plain, dairy-free
- 1 tsp. of vanilla extract, pure

For frosting:

- 1 cup of shortening, palm
- 1/4 cup of syrup, maple
- 2 tsp. of vanilla extract, pure
- 2 tbsp. of flour, arrow root
- 1/2 tsp. of gelatin, grass-fed, unflavored
- 8 oz. of melted, cooled chocolate chips, semi-sweet

Directions:

1. Preheat oven to 350F.

2. Place baking soda, coconut flour and sea salt in small bowl. Whisk and combine.

3. Whisk 8 oz. of chocolate, vanilla extract, yogurt, eggs and maple syrup in medium sized bowl.

4. Whisk in coconut flour mixture till smooth. Allow batter to sit for 8-10 minutes.

5. Pour batter in two x 9" cake pans. Bake for 18-22 minutes. Cool for 8-10 minutes and place on cooling rack.

6. Place palm shortening, melted chocolate, gelatin, arrow root, vanilla extract and syrup in standing mixer bowl. Whisk for 2-3 minutes till fluffy and light.

7. For assembly, place one layer cake on plate. Top with 1/3 of frosting.

8. Put second layer on the top and use the rest of the frosting to frost remainder of cake. Serve.

Conclusion

Here we are at the end of Nature's Recipe Grain Free Cookbook. These 30 Deliciously Easy Grain Free Recipes were intended to Keep You Known for Tasty Yet Healthy Treats. I hope that you were able to enjoy preparing all 30 recipes and that your family and loved ones are excited about a healthier, grain free lifestyle.

Please take a few minutes to share your thoughts and feedback on the platform on which you purchased the book. Then continue to mix and match recipes until you have mastered all thirty.

Enjoy!

Printed in Great Britain
by Amazon